Exhausted!

A PSYCHOLOGIST'S GUIDE TO DEALING WITH
CHRONIC FATIGUE

Dr Catherine Sykes

Dedication

I dedicate this book to Dr Emee Estacio for her ongoing encouragement and support. Her insights into publishing were a crucial factor in getting this book finished. She really is a star! (http://www.thepamecode.com)

Contents

Discover how to feel energised to lead a life with purpose.

Are you exhausted all the time? Do you try your best to get plenty of sleep but still feel exhausted when you wake up or do you find it hard to sleep despite feeling exhausted? Do you feel that the days are just passing and nothing is changing in your life? Do you worry that you will always be like this? Perhaps you have tried numerous methods and read lots of books, perhaps even tried a range of diets to help you feel a little more energised. You may be experiencing chronic fatigue, your regular state is just exhausted and has been for a very long time.

Nowadays, the number of people experiencing feelings of constant fatigue severe enough to impact their daily lives is increasing. This is often accompanied by regular periods of getting sick or having some kind of minor ailments. For some, this takes them down the road to a diagnosis of Chronic Fatigue Syndrome (CFS).

The symptoms of fatigue and CFS can be distressing, and it can be a lonely experience. I'm passionate about empowering people to improve their quality of life using psychological techniques, such as Cognitive Behaviour Therapy (CBT), Acceptance Commitment Therapy (ACT) and Somatic Psychology. If your CFS has a physical component, I do not claim to be able to cure you. However, psychological therapies can help to strengthen the body-mind connection and work to address some of the emotional and social factors that are part-and-parcel of ongoing fatigue and CFS. Such therapies can improve your quality of life and lead a purposeful life.

This book is specially written to help both those who suffer with frequent feelings of fatigue without a diagnosis and for those who have been diagnosed with CFS. From my experience, there are various common psychological components associated with CFS and long-term chronic fatigue that has not been diagnosed as CFS. I will examine these components in more detail later in this book. I have worked with many people who have come to see me in my private clinic for depression who are also fatigued all the time who have eventually gone on to receive a diagnosis of CFS. I have decided to write this book as I think it is important to take seriously the increase in acceptance of being exhausted all the time. It has become acceptable to reply "I'm busy" or "I'm exhausted" when asked "how are you?" It is not a normal state of being. It is an unhealthy state, that from my experience of working privately with thousands of clients, can be part of a trajectory to CFS. It is a state that takes you further away from your life's purpose.

It is important to note that those with a diagnosis of CFS may have different disease pathways such as a virus or an immunological abnormality. Understanding the pathophysiology of CFS is beyond the remit of this book. You should always consult with your doctor before making any changes to your routine and activity levels.

In my practice as a Psychologist, I have seen a marked increase in the number of people with a CFS diagnosis and people who are constantly exhausted. I am not saying that these two groups experience the same severity of fatigue, but there are common ways to help both groups cope and manage the exhaustion. I will discuss these coping mechanisms later on in the book.

WHAT DOES FATIGUE FEEL LIKE?

If you suffer from fatigue on a regular basis, it can sometimes be hard to describe how you are feeling to other people. However, these feelings can have a real impact on your energy levels, productivity and overall mood and enjoyment of life. Sufferers can also experience problems socially, as it can be hard for others to fully understand how your fatigue affects you. Unfortunately, if you have CFS, the causes of many of the unpleasant symptoms are not yet fully understood, and it can be extremely frustrating to not fully understand why you are feeling this way. However, these symptoms are very real and are not simply 'in your head'. Here are some of the most common symptoms:

- Fatigue: A feeling of extreme tiredness and exhaustion that interrupts or prevents you carrying out your day-to-day tasks. Fatigue is not simply 'feeling tired', despite common misconceptions of the condition. It is a sensation of exhaustion that goes far beyond the sensation of tiredness that most people feel after a long day at work or a tough workout. You may feel physically fatigued, where your exhaustion is felt in your body. Your muscles may feel weak and you have constant aches in your body. Also, you may feel mentally fatigued, finding it hard to focus or engage in tasks involving thinking. People suffering from fatigue or with a definitive CFS diagnosis may suffer from either physical or mental fatigue, but many suffer from both. These feelings can be debilitating. While well-meaning but ill-informed people may advise you to 'get a good night's sleep', chronic fatigue does not resolve itself this way. Even after good-quality sleep, CFS sufferers still wake up feeling fatigued and exhausted.

- Malaise: This is a feeling of overwhelming exhaustion and weakness. It also gives a sensation of general discomfort, like the symptoms you experience when you are suffering from an infection or virus. Many people who suffer from ongoing fatigue or CFS experience an intense feeling of malaise following physical activity. For some people, this occurs after taking part in exercise, but for many sufferers even carrying out day-to-day tasks, such as taking a shower or doing light housework, can result in debilitating exhaustion. This can last upwards of 24 hours and can be extremely unpleasant and distressing to experience. This phenomenon is referred to as Post-Exertional Malaise in CFS sufferers, or PEM for short. Unfortunately, some doctors still do not acknowledge that PEM exists. This can be highly frustrating if your feelings of malaise have been written off as just feeling 'tired'. Some patients may even have been told that their PEM is a way of avoiding exerting themselves physically. This is unfair and incorrect, and you should be reassured that research is now showing that very real physiological problems are often the root cause of PEM. As anyone without CFS will tell you, feeling completely wiped out after even intense exercise is not a common experience unless there is a cause.

- Headaches: A common complaint for CFS sufferers is recurring and stubborn headaches without an identifiable cause. Unfortunately, the cause of this pain is still not completely understood by doctors, but it is a very real and unpleasant symptom of CFS. Long-term pain can cause low mood and make life miserable. You deserve to have your pain taken seriously by your medical care provider.

- Sleep disturbance: Problems with sleep are common in CFS sufferers and those who suffer from fatigue but who are yet to be formally diagnosed. If you suffer from fatigue, it's likely that you experience episodes of sleepiness during the day when other people feel wide awake. Also, people with CFS often struggle to fall asleep or stay asleep throughout the night, even if they feel completely exhausted and ready to nod off. Another common issue is a sensation of waking up unrefreshed, even if you have slept deeply for a long time. These feelings can be very distressing and get in the way of your day-to-day activities. Unfortunately, like so many aspects of CFS, the causes of these problems are not fully understood. This can lead to feelings of frustration, especially if you feel like your sleep problems are not being taken seriously by people around you.

- Difficulties with concentration: People with ongoing fatigue or CFS often find concentrating on tasks very difficult. Other areas of thinking, such as memory, can also be affected. Many people describe this as a feeling of having a 'foggy head', and it can be extremely troubling if you do a job that requires a lot of mental agility. The feeling of not being able to recall information can be really distressing, but it is a frequent symptom that comes along with CFS. These symptoms may be worsened if you are also suffering from sleep disturbances.

- Muscle pain: Sore muscles and joints are very common complaints amongst CFS sufferers, and the level of pain can vary from mild to severe pain that impacts your quality of life. Some people also find that they get recurrent sore throats, as if they have a throat infection, but without the accompanying illness. Often, there is no redness, swelling or inflammation visible at the point of pain, but this does not mean that the pain you are experiencing is not real.

In this book, I will use the terms exhausted, fatigue and CFS interchangeably. If you don't have a diagnosis of CFS and, having read through the description of CFS symptoms, you are concerned that you may be suffering from it, you should consult a doctor to assess your symptoms. Your doctor will probably look to see if you have four or more of the following symptoms: sore throat, lymph node pain, muscle pain, joint pain, post-exertional malaise, headaches, memory and concentration difficulties, and unrefreshing sleep. In addition to these symptoms, your doctor will assess whether the fatigue is alleviated by rest, and whether it is impacting on occupational, social or educational activities. To confirm diagnosis, the symptoms must have lasted longer than six months with no other organic cause found.

If you already have a diagnosis, it is important to continue to follow your doctor's advice in addition to the guidance in this book.

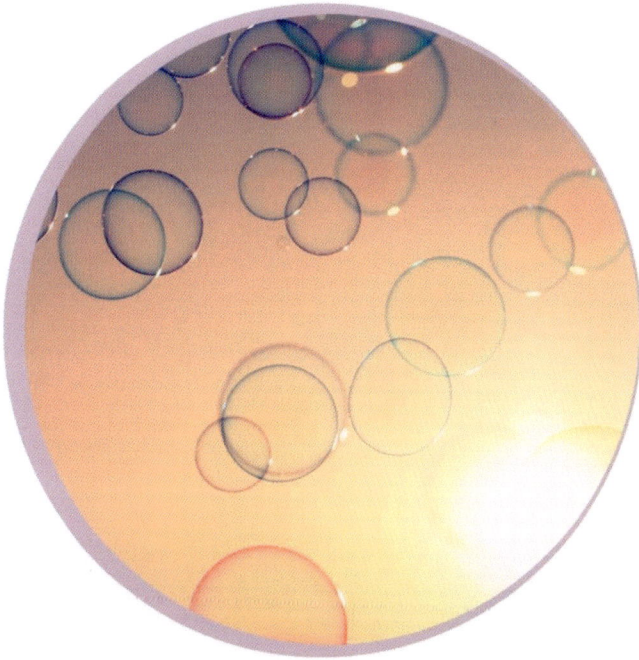

Causes

Unfortunately, for those suffering from CFS, the causes of the condition are not fully understood yet. For this reason, there isn't a medical testing process to diagnose CFS in sufferers. Instead, doctors have to diagnose CFS from the symptoms experienced by the patient. However, there are some theories about what events could trigger CFS. The most mainstream theories are that CFS is a complication following a **viral infection** and/or that it is triggered by a period of intense **psychological stress**. For some sufferers, the symptoms they experience may be caused by a permanent physiological component which cannot be cured using psychological techniques. However, the emotional and social impact of living with CFS can, for some people, be eased by working with a psychologist to develop coping strategies and mechanisms and to gain a deeper understanding of your own fatigue and energy levels.

The psychological stress that triggers chronic fatigue may be a significant life event that is obvious such as a divorce or a home building project. For some, it is several life events and stressors that all collide at the same time. It can also be a very busy lifestyle in which you are constantly pushing yourself close to your limits. Many people lead busy lives, but some people spend months on end without taking any breaks during the day and work late into the night. Occasionally our bodies can handle busy periods but when it becomes a permanent lifestyle, our bodies struggle. Some people turn to other unhealthy habits such as drinking alcohol on a regular basis or eating quick processed foods to help cope with the lifestyle. Sometimes this fast pace is followed by days of rest or hardly doing anything. This leads to a 'boom and bust' pattern of activity in which the body is constantly being pushed close or beyond its limits followed by intense periods of rest. This irregular pace of life can be confusing for the bodies and upset its natural bodily rhythms.

Alongside this busy 'boom and bust' lifestyle, there are the **emotional** aspects of life. Quite often it is an over-conscientious mindset and a maladaptive perfectionist thinking style that contribute to and maintain a 'boom and bust' lifestyle. Always wanting to do and be the best in every situation can put unrealistic demands on your mind and body leading to worry and anxiety and ultimately low mood. All of these physical, social and emotional factors lead to symptoms of fatigue which can then lead to sleep problems, loss of fitness and loss of muscle strength which can then lead to a worsening of symptoms.

Then the worry about the symptoms can lead some people to **increase their focus on the symptoms**. They become hypervigilant, constantly checking their body and their symptoms. The problem is that hypervigilance puts the mind and body on alert which interferes with our ability to accurately interpret the significance of the symptoms. The hypervigilance and perfectionist mindset can then lead to **increased attempts to find a cure**. This is understandable as it is not pleasant to be so fatigued all the time. However, the perfectionist mindset can go onto overdrive, looking for cures, being impatient when no immediate or not enough results are found, then quickly switching to another cure or therapy, getting depressed and frustrated in the process as it may seem like nothing is working, this can lead to a feeling of hopelessness and a **sense of loss of control** which results in a **reduction of activity**. Before long, the perfectionist creeps back in and starts looking for more cures. This pattern keeps the individual in a 'boom and bust' pattern of recovery and state of alert and anxiety and depression which overtime can worsen the symptoms.

This image is available at:

https://www.zenitudeselfhelp.com

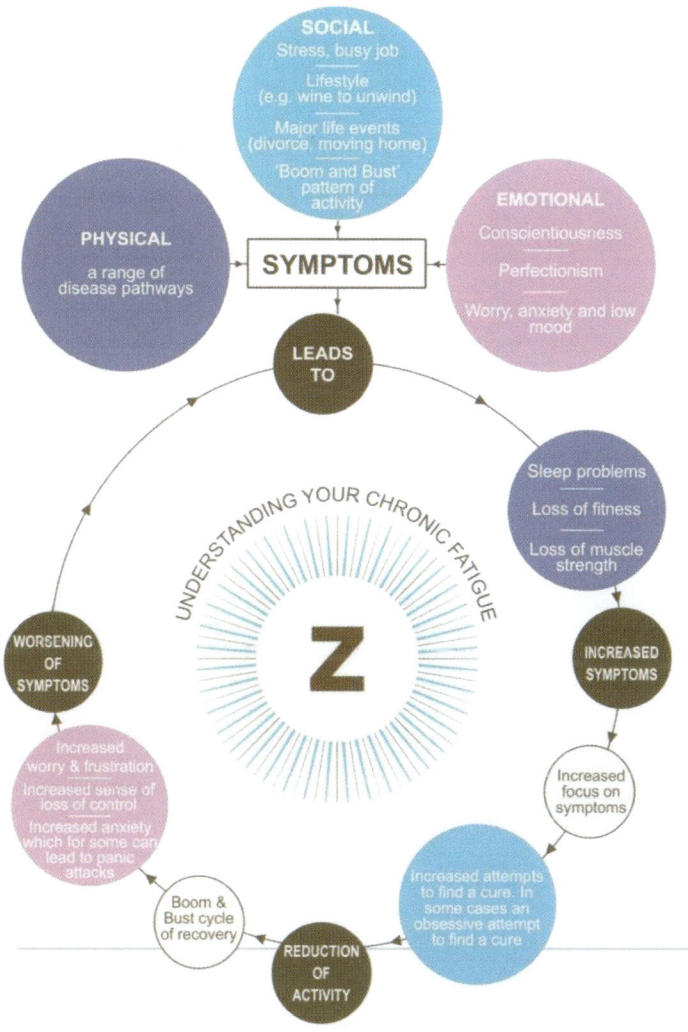

SOCIAL
Stress, busy job

Lifestyle
(e.g. wine to unwind)

Major life events
(divorce, moving home)

'Boom and Bust'
pattern of
activity

PHYSICAL
a range of
disease pathways

SYMPTOMS

EMOTIONAL
Conscientiousness

Perfectionism

Worry, anxiety and low
mood

LEADS
TO

UNDERSTANDING YOUR CHRONIC FATIGUE

Z

Sleep problems

Loss of fitness

Loss of muscle
strength

WORSENING
OF
SYMPTOMS

INCREASED
SYMPTOMS

Increased
worry & frustration

Increased sense of
loss of control

Increased anxiety
which for some can
lead to panic
attacks

Increased
focus on
symptoms

Boom &
Bust cycle
of recovery

Increased attempts
to find a cure. In
some cases an
obsessive attempt
to find a cure

REDUCTION
OF
ACTIVITY

IS COGNITIVE BEHAVIOUR THERAPY THE RIGHT TREATMENT FOR CFS?

Cognitive Behaviour Therapy for Chronic Fatigue Syndrome has received bad press recently, as it is claimed that some researchers may have exaggerated the benefits. Unfortunately, we live in a world where even scientists need to market themselves and make big claims to justify spending large amounts of public money. Sometimes, it is not even the scientists who are making the big claims. Often, the press makes outlandish and sweeping statements about all sorts of health-related matters in order to attract readers.

Science is political and it can get personal. Sadly, this bad press has discouraged many people living with CFS from undertaking Cognitive Behaviour Therapy. I do think this is a shame, as I have helped many clients with a range of fatigue levels and disease pathways to better manage chronic fatigue. Not in all cases, but for many, their symptoms have disappeared, and they have returned to a normal life. I suspect the fact that there are differing disease pathways will contribute to the varying degrees of outcomes. Despite the controversy, I do believe that Cognitive Behaviour Therapy can play a role in helping people manage fatigue. I left academia several years ago, so

I make this statement as a private practitioner who has witnessed the benefits. The advantages of being a private practitioner mean that I don't get sucked into the politics of research. I also believe combining another branch of psychology called Somatic Psychology can play a role in helping people deal with fatigue.

In this book, I draw upon theories from Cognitive Behaviour Therapy and Somatic Psychology. Somatic Psychology appeals to me, as it acknowledges the body as a source of wisdom and information. I think, in this busy world of abundance and reduced boundaries, it has become easy to lose the mind–body connection and to mindlessly push our bodies to their limits. Research shows that supporting people with CFS to identify their values can be beneficial for long-term management of their condition. This is why I think the use of Acceptance Commitment Therapy (ACT) is useful for managing long-term fatigue. I think this is particularly useful for people who have experienced an unexpected stressful life event. Quite often, the shock of the event can cause a 'freeze' reaction or a psychological sense of being 'stuck' or 'hit by a brick wall'. Suddenly, the person's usual ways of coping are no longer useful. Similarly, maladaptive perfectionism can lead to a paralysis of activity as the self-enforced expectations are so strong and unrealistic that any action feels problematic. A new direction and new ways of coping are needed.

What will you gain from this book?

There are several potential benefits from reading this book:

1. More purpose in your life.
2. The best use of energy levels.
3. Prevention of your symptoms worsening or becoming disabling.
4. An ability to cope with the social and emotional impact of living with fatigue.
5. An understanding of the mind-body connection to give you the best possible circumstances for recovery.

As you journey through the stages of the book, you will find yourself developing a greater awareness, understanding and appreciation of your body. This includes observing your symptoms and learning what they mean for you as an individual. You will learn to view your symptoms as useful and important warning signs that your body is sending you, and which should be responded to. Ignoring these 'signals' from your body, such as fatigue, can lead to activity-induced worsening of your condition and can prevent natural recovery. However, too much focus on your symptoms can also lead to activity avoidance and low mood. You will learn how to respond to your body's signals in a positive and helpful way.

As part of this process, you will learn to plan your activities in a way that creates the ideal balance with resting periods. The aim is to help you maximize what you can achieve whilst keeping activity at a level that doesn't cause worsening of your symptoms.

HOW TO USE THIS BOOK

Ideally, it's a great idea to purchase a special notebook to use while you progress through the book. This is the perfect way to jot down useful ideas and notes and to celebrate progress whilst engaging the problem-solving parts of your brain. However, many people nowadays are in the habit of making electronic notes on their phones or other devices. If this is true for you, now is not the time to try and break the habit. While hand-written notes are better, any way of recording your thoughts, feelings and progress will provide benefits.

Your diary is a really important part of this process, so it's important that you use it in a way that's manageable and sustainable. The notes you make don't need to be extensive, but should be made in a way that's both helpful and manageable over the length of the process. So, be realistic with your expectations of yourself regarding your diary entries. It's far better to write concise notes every day than to write an essay in the first few days and then stop because it's unsustainable.

If you're new to keeping diaries or journals, it can be hard at first to get into the habit. If you have never kept one before, it's all too easy to forget to make your daily entry. For this reason, I recommend that you set yourself an alarm or reminder on a device until you've established the habit of writing.

As part of my practice, I often work with clients who experience very severe fatigue. The benefits of face-to-face support and encouragement cannot be underestimated, and of course you don't get this with a book. For this reason, it's a great idea to ask a family member or friend to provide support and encouragement throughout the process. Ask your chosen person to read this book beforehand and agree with them the type and frequency of support you require to make sure they are able to provide it.

This book is designed to be easy to follow and guides you through 4 phases that will take you to leading a energized life with purpose. The 4 phases are important steps. Making any change is not easy. As humans, we naturally go to the familiar. It is safer and easier. Phase 1 will help you to get motivated to make some change. Please don't be tempted to skip it and get straight to the making changes in Phases 2 and 3. If you have any difficulties with making changes, keep coming back to Phase 1. Finally Phase 4 helps you to think about maintaining your changes so you can lead your energized life with purpose. You can take all of the Phases at your own pace.

To help make this as clear as possible, there are two icons to look out for:

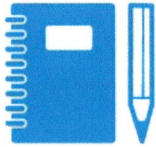

When you see this icon, it is time to PAUSE and write notes in your notebook or create a note in your phone, tablet or eBook. If you are in a busy environment, close your eyes and think about the questions before you take notes.

This icon is to let you know that it's time to set a reminder on your phone or on a sticky note.

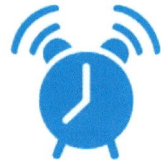

Phase 1 – Motivation and seeing the end in mind

Time to get out your notebook or noting device. Please leave the first few pages blank for an exercise later in the book.

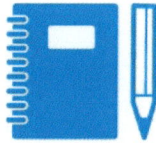

When did fatigue become a problem for you? What was going on in your life? Can you remember an incident that could have been a trigger for you? What was your reaction to this incident?

During this exercise, try to take yourself back to the time when you first noticed fatigue having an impact on your day-to-day life. For many people, CFS first becomes noticeable when they have spent a prolonged period of time functioning at an activity intensity close to the limit of what they can cope with, often paying much more attention to others than themselves. This can continue for some time, with the person becoming more and more tired and burnt-out, and putting more and more unrealistic expectations upon themselves. Usually, periods of over-vigorous activity are followed by a long period of extended rest and reduced activities. This is because the limit for what the person can cope with has been lowered. After a while, the person may begin to feel better, prompting them to resume an unmanageable level of activity, despite their limit now being lowered.

This can become a cycle, where the person engages in overly high levels of activity and then 'crashes', requiring extended rest periods, which can make the problem worse in the long term, as it is difficult to establish any kind of routine. At some stage, the person reaches a point that feels like 'the final straw', where they can no longer continue to function in this way. This is a scary place to find yourself. When we are scared, our reaction can be to escape to seek safety rather than to deal with the actual causes.

For others, a particular event is the trigger, like a viral infection or a very stressful life event, such as the loss of a loved one, a divorce, being bullied, being severely let down by someone you thought you could trust, an unexpected life event or a traumatic event. At such times, our reaction can be one of surprise. When we are surprised, we tend to stop. The purpose of stopping is to reorient yourself. Without support or guidance, some people remain in stop mode, as they have not processed the event and have not worked out the next step.

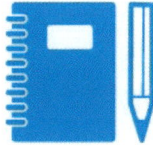

What were your feelings and emotions during the time that you first became fatigued? List them and rate the intensity of the emotion from 1-10, with 1 being hardly and 10 being extremely.

If you can't remember any feelings, ask yourself how someone might feel if they were experiencing what you were going through. Use the Wheel of Emotions, which is based on Dr Robert Plutchik's proposal that we have eight primary emotions that serve as the foundation of all emotions. Learning to identify and name your primary emotion and the combination of emotions can be very empowering.

https://www.zenitudeselfhelp.com

WHEEL OF EMOTIONS

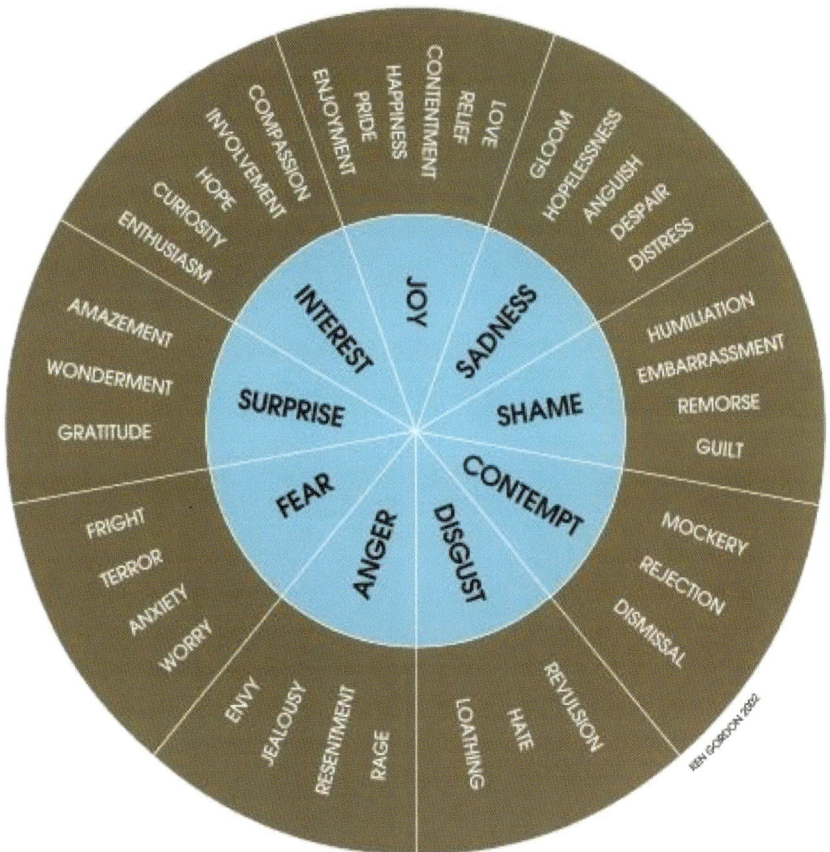

The ideal end goal of the process is to gain an acceptance of your limits and to set a meaningful routine where you can balance activity and rest in a way that suits your personal circumstances, symptoms and values, breaking the 'boom and bust' cycle and knowing where you want to take your life. In order to move into the future, you will need to accept the past and let go of the intense negative feelings.

List the emotions that you rated above 7 in intensity.

Now, get a piece of paper or start an electronic note. Start to write a description of your circumstances during this initial period of fatigue, weave these intense emotions into the description. Use the first person, I, to describe your story. It may take several attempts to write your descriptions. That's okay, just notice any difficulties you experience as you try to write, notice your emotions, notice what you do. Do you avoid writing, do you get up to eat something, do you sit still and feel blocked? Whatever happens for you, notice it, allow it in, does it give you any additional information about yourself, then commit to writing, even if only a few words at first. Start to write.

Once you have written your description, read it and re-read it. Ask yourself if you would like to share your description with someone you trust. You don't have to but it may help to share a sense of vulnerability with someone you trust. The sense of connection you receive from sharing a vulnerability can be very powerful. It can be the beginning of a healing process.

When you have finished your description, leave it for a few days, then go back to it and ask yourself if you are ready to let it go. Keep doing this until the answer is yes. Then, find a way to destroy the description. If it is paper, you can tear it up, burn it or maybe even send it into the sea or a river or a stream. Ask yourself what feels appropriate. Some people find it useful to have a 'Good-bye Ceremony' in which the description is peacefully acknowledged and sent away. If you have written an electronic note, your option is to delete it, but you can think about different settings in which you want to press delete. As you destroy or delete your description, say the following:

"You belong to the past, you no longer have any power over me, I'm letting you go".

BONUS MATERIAL

To enhance your sensation of letting go, I have prepared an exercise that enables you to tune into the physical sensation of letting go. By listening to the short audio file on a regular basis, your body will become familiar with the physical sensation of letting go and will be more able to recognize when you are tense.

Download at Zenitudeselfhelp.com

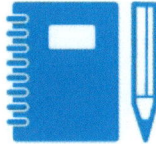

Pause and think, what would managing your fatigue look like in an ideal world?

How do you want to feel? What will your life look like if you are less fatigued? What will you be doing?

Once you have completed this task, take a closer look at your ideas and aspirations and ask yourself: is this realistic given my personal circumstances? It is very important that this image belongs to you and your life circumstances. If it includes any 'shoulds' and 'musts', this is probably not your own personal realistic vision. If it is not realistic, pause and think again. Knowing what your values are in life will help you to make this vision your own and reorient you to a future that is based on your values, which may have changed after a stressful life event.

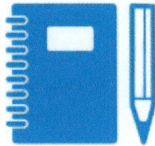

What are your values?

Values are your deepest wishes for how you want to behave as a human being. Values are not about what you want to obtain or achieve; they are about how you want to behave or act on an ongoing basis. Understanding why you are busy or why you want to recover is very important. Having a purpose makes it that bit easier to endure a difficulty or make difficult changes.

There are hundreds of different values, and below you'll find a list of some common ones suggested by Russ Harris, the author of 'The Happiness Trap'. All these values are good values to have, but I want you to focus on you personally and what is important to you. There are no such things as 'right values' or 'wrong values'. Similarly, your values may differ from another person's values. So, read through the list below and write a letter next to each value: V = Very important, Q = Quite important, and N = Not so important. Try to score *about ten* of them as *Very important*. Some people find this exercise difficult as they find that all of the values are important. All of the values are important but try to focus on what is really very important to you personally.

1. Acceptance: to be open to and accepting of myself, others, life etc.

2. Adventure: to be adventurous; to actively seek, create, or explore novel or stimulating experiences

3. Assertiveness: to respectfully stand up for my rights and request what I want

4. Authenticity: to be authentic, genuine, and real; to be true to myself

5. Beauty: to appreciate, create, nurture, or cultivate beauty in myself, others, the environment etc.

6. Caring: to be caring towards myself, others, the environment etc.

7. Challenge: to keep challenging myself to grow, learn, and improve

8. Compassion: to act with kindness towards those who are suffering

9. Connection: to engage fully in whatever I am doing, and be fully present with others

10. Contribution: to contribute, help, assist, or make a positive difference to myself or others

11. Conformity: to be respectful and obedient of rules and obligations

12. Cooperation: to be cooperative and collaborative with others

13. Courage: to be courageous or brave; to persist in the face of fear, threat, or difficulty

14. Creativity: to be creative or innovative

15. Curiosity: to be curious, open-minded, and interested; to explore and discover

16. Encouragement: to encourage and reward behaviour that I value in myself or others

17. Equality: to treat others as equal to myself, and vice-versa

18. Excitement: to seek, create, and engage in activities that are exciting, stimulating, or thrilling

19. Fairness: to be fair to myself or others

20. Fitness: to maintain or improve my fitness; to look after my physical and mental health and wellbeing

21. Flexibility: to adjust and adapt readily to changing circumstances

22. Freedom: to live freely; to choose how I live and behave, or help others to do likewise

23. Friendliness: to be friendly, companionable, or agreeable towards others

24. Forgiveness: to be forgiving towards myself or others

25. Fun: to be fun-loving; to seek, create, and engage in fun-filled activities

26. Generosity: to be generous, sharing, and giving to myself or others

27. Gratitude: to be grateful for and appreciative of the positive aspects of myself, others, and life

28. Honesty: to be honest, truthful, and sincere with myself and others

29. Humour: to see and appreciate the humorous side of life

30. Humility: to be humble or modest; to let my achievements speak for themselves

31. Industry: to be industrious, hard-working, and dedicated

32. Independence: to be self-supportive, and choose my own way of doing things

33. Intimacy: to open up, reveal, and share myself -- emotionally or physically – in my close personal relationships

34. Justice: to uphold justice and fairness

35. Kindness: to be kind, compassionate, considerate, nurturing, or caring towards myself or others

36. Love: to act lovingly or affectionately towards myself or others

37. Mindfulness: to be conscious of, open to, and curious about my here-and-now experience

38. Order: to be orderly and organised

39. Open-mindedness: to think things through, see things from other's points of view, and weigh evidence fairly

40. Patience: to wait calmly for what I want

41. Persistence: to continue resolutely, despite problems or difficulties

42. Power: to strongly influence or wield authority over others, e.g. taking charge, leading, organising

43. Reciprocity: to build relationships in which there is a fair balance of giving and taking

44. Respect: to be respectful towards myself or others; to be polite, considerate, and to show positive regard

45. Responsibility: to be responsible and accountable for my actions

46. Romance: to be romantic; to display and express love or strong affection

47. Safety: to secure, protect, or ensure the safety of myself or others

48. Self-awareness: to be aware of my own thoughts, feelings, and actions

49. Self-care: to look after my health and wellbeing, and ensure my needs are met

50. Self-development: to keep growing, advancing, or improving in knowledge, skills, character, or life experience

51. Self-control: to act in accordance with my own ideals

52. Sensuality: to create, explore, and enjoy experiences that stimulate the five senses

53. Sexuality: to explore or express my sexuality

54. Spirituality: to connect with things bigger than myself

55. Skilfulness: to continually practice and improve my skills, and apply myself fully when using them

56. Supportiveness: to be supportive, helpful, encouraging, and available to myself or others

57. Trust: to be trustworthy; to be loyal, faithful, sincere, and reliable

58. Insert your own unlisted value(s) here: *Financial Stability & Independen*

59. Once you have marked each value as V, Q, N, go through all the Vs and select the top six that are the most important to you.

connection   intimacy
friendliness   gratitude
love & romance self development & control
spirituality   self care of health
balance
safety
financial
    safety.

60. Finally, write down these values in your notebook
on the first pages.

Set a reminder in your phone to remind you of your 6
values on a daily basis for 1 month, then every other day for
the next month, then weekly for a month then finally set a
reminder of your values every month.

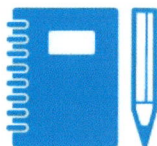

Once you are happy with your chosen values and are
satisfied that your vision is realistic, imagine the physical
sensations you would feel if this vision became a reality.

List the feelings you would expect from your vision.

Using your notes, try to create a symbol of this positive and
realistic future in your mind. The type of symbol you
choose is personal and could be a visual image, words or
even a sound. It should include images of the end vision,
but also images of the process of getting to the end vision.

For example, I worked with a client who wanted to
interact more with her children. Her symbol was the image
of a water slide. She could hear the sounds of lots of

children in a frenzy of joy. She could feel the water on her body and could focus on the sensation of rapid movement. Her process involved asking a friend to take her children swimming while she watched them play. Then it involved going into the changing rooms with her children. The next image involved her in the swimming pool with her friend and her children, followed by her in the swimming pool alone with her children, then taking the slide with her children.

Try to visualise, hear, and engage with your meaningful symbol as regularly as possible. This will quickly prime your mind to focus on what you do want. Our mind likes images. Images of what we do want make change a little easier.

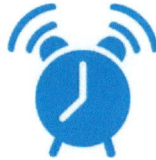

Set a reminder to take time every day to direct your focus onto your symbol and practice the quick and simple exercise described below.

Take several energetic breaths while imagining your symbol for your future. Focusing on your breathing doesn't need to be complicated or stressful. Just pause and become aware of your breathing. Close your eyes if you wish. What words would you use to describe your breathing? What movement do you need to take to give that breath just a little more energy?

This might take some time to practice. Tuning into your symbol of your vision should help your breathing to feel more energetic. Become familiar with this energetic sensation, even if you can only hold it for a few seconds. With practice, you will be able to hold this energetic breath for longer.

Try to stay with your symbol of your future for 15-20 seconds.

Plan when in your day you can tune into this future self. Where will you be when you access this image of your future self?

Making time to focus on this symbol of your future is an important and motivating step towards making it a reality. Set a reminder on your phone or in your diary to tune into and connect to your future self and your meaningful symbol every day.

To enhance your visualization process, you can print an image to stick at the front of your notebook, or add a photo to the notes section in your phone, or use the photo as a screen saver. Some people also like to create a secret board on Pinterest with images of all the stages of progress towards their vision.

Phase 2 – What's going on for you? Becoming in tune with your body and mind and obtaining your own data

Phase 2 of the process is about becoming more in tune with the body-mind connection and making links between what you do and how you feel. During this phase, you will need to write in your notebook and use a structured diary, which can be found at the end of Phase 2. This diary will be a very important tool to help you better understand the link between your body and mind. The diary is a great way to capture data about your fatigue, activity levels and feelings, and will help you to develop a greater level of self-awareness and the ability to self-monitor. It is important though that you don't become too obsessed about using the diary. I would suggest a maximum period of 1 month for recording in your diary.

This is the first vital step towards the 'future you' that you visualized in Phase 1 and will help you to self-regulate. Before you start using your diary, it's important to gain a deeper understanding of why listening to your body and mind is so important and to gain some insight into some of the factors that cause fatigue.

By paying attention to how your body feels, you are tapping into a wealth of information and wisdom about your health. There is an important relationship between how you think, what you do, and how your body feels. By listening to your body and making notes in your diary, you will start to notice objective patterns between your behaviour and your symptoms. This may feel strange at first. Many people are not use to really living in their body. Their experience of living mainly comes from a sense of being in their head. This is particularly true for people with a perfectionist mindset. Their head rules their existence. Perfectionism has become a way to feel safe. I ask you not to dismiss the paying attention to your body aspect of this book. This can help you to start taking positive steps towards self-regulation and allows you to regain a sense of control.

Think carefully about what it feels like when you are experiencing sensations of fatigue. You can think about the physical symptoms and emotional feelings associated with fatigue.

Try to note down some of the words that you feel best describe your fatigue.

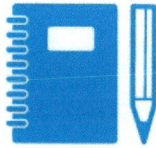

Also, try to distinguish what type of fatigue you experience most regularly. There are two main types of fatigue that people with CFS commonly experience:

- Burnt-out fatigue: This type of fatigue is associated with feeling like you've done too much activity or at too high an intensity.
- Rust-out fatigue: Conversely, rust-out fatigue is the feeling of not having done enough. This can give you the sensation of feeling stagnant, stuck or 'rusty'.

If you have found yourself stuck in the 'boom and bust' cycle I described at the beginning of the book, you may experience both types of fatigue at different times. You may feel the 'burnt-out' fatigue during your periods of over-activity and the 'rust-out' fatigue after extended periods of rest.

Next, think carefully about any factors that affect the intensity of your symptoms. Already you will probably be able to think of certain activities or behaviours that result in a worsening of your symptoms such as spending too much time socializing, going to a particular place, driving, sitting at home all day. However, it's also a good idea to ask yourself if there is anything that makes your symptoms better such as when you see a certain friend or when someone is not at home.

SUBSTANCES THAT AFFECT YOUR SYMPTOMS

Many people who suffer from fatigue find that they struggle to get quality sleep, or that they don't feel refreshed even after sleeping for long periods. Quite often, unresolved worries prevent people from having a deep, refreshing sleep. However, there are substances present in many people's lifestyles that can have a negative effect on sleep quality. The most common are alcohol, nicotine and caffeine. Some medications can also make it harder to fall or stay asleep.

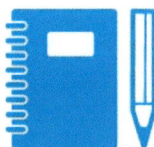

It may seem too simple to think about substances that affect your symptoms. I do always like to start with paying attention to simple observations. Ask yourself what your typical habits are when it comes to these substances, and whether you take any medications that could be interfering with your sleep. Jot down any thoughts in your notebook.

THINKING ABOUT FATIGUE

It may sound counter-intuitive to examine the way you think about fatigue. Taking time to try and gain a deeper understanding of how you think about your fatigue does not mean it is all in your head; quite the opposite. Just like any other illness, the way we cope with our symptoms and feelings can impact the way we experience the illness positively or negatively. Therefore, taking time to examine your thinking process is a valuable tool when it comes to managing fatigue. So, ask yourself the question: how do I think about fatigue? Here are some key points to consider regarding how you think and feel about your fatigue.

HOW DO YOU THINK YOU SHOULD COPE WITH FATIGUE?

An important factor to consider at this stage is how you think you should be coping with your fatigue. Sometimes, we can develop beliefs about coping with fatigue that may not necessarily be productive or positive. Here are some common thoughts about coping with CFS:

- The best way to respond to feeling fatigued is to reduce activity levels or avoid activity altogether.
- Exercise is bound to result in pain or discomfort.
- Scheduling rest periods into the day is unacceptable

and a waste of time.

- Symptoms are a sign that some kind of damage is being done.
- I need to carefully pay attention to my symptoms in order to better manage them.
- I must always do my very best in every way possible to manage my fatigue.
- I've done my best and it is not working.
- What's the point? Maybe I should just accept that I'm going to be like this forever.
- Why can't I fix this?
- I'm getting so much support and I'm not getting better.
- I must get an appointment with (expert X). It worked for Y.
- Maybe I should try…..

Another key question to ask yourself is how much time you spend worrying about your fatigue or whether you are coping with it in the right way. Through worrying, do you usually find solutions to your concerns? Jot down any thoughts that come out of this line of thinking.

As with any long-term condition, it can be all too easy to fall into a vicious cycle of unhelpful thoughts and behaviours. While these can become deeply ingrained, they can be changed! Using strategies such as CBT can help to retrain you into more productive ways of thinking and behaving.

There are two common ways in which people living with CFS often fall into vicious cycles. The first is by developing unhelpful illness beliefs or fears, where you find yourself thinking about your fatigue in ways which cause excessive worry, frustration, guilt or lead to a fear of activity, which ultimately lead to either:

1. a 'freeze' response in which you try to accept the fatigue and don't do anything further to facilitate recovery. In this state, you deliberately avoid activity altogether for fear of making your fatigue worse.

2. If you suffer from fatigue, experiencing pain or increased exhaustion after physical or mental exertion is probably all too familiar. Naturally, this can lead you

3. to worry that you are doing yourself some harm by participating in your day-to-day activities. A logical solution to this appears to be to avoid activity

altogether and to rest for long periods of time. However, prolonged rest can actually slow your recovery by reducing your limit for tolerating activity and lowering your all-round physical fitness.

4. Avoiding any sort of activity for fear of making your symptoms worse can impact your life in other ways beyond the physical. Stopping your day-to-day activities on a daily basis can cause you to lose confidence in your ability to do them. For example, you may stop socialising with particular friends, managing your home or doing exercise that you used to enjoy. This can also lead to increased social isolation and lowered mood, and the thought of starting up these activities again can provoke anxiety and lead to more avoidance.

OR

5. A 'fight' response which results in you over-trying in the recovery process and gives a sense that you are in a battle with your own body. It is good to take your condition seriously and to actively try methods to improve it. However, I find that some people can become too pre-occupied with searching and trying different remedies to the point that it becomes an exhausting activity. Also, what happens is that people

become so desperate to find a cure that they don't give the solutions they are trying a fair chance. They become easily frustrated by the lack of progress with a chosen method, then quickly move to the next option. The searching, pre-occupation, the efforts to carry out the chosen method and the frustration can compound any existing fatigue.

Below are examples of the draining emotions, such as worry, frustration, guilt, and shame, that follow certain thoughts about coping.

Coping Thoughts	Resulting Draining Emotions
'Why can't I fix this?'	Frustration, Guilt, Worry.
'I'm getting so much support and I'm not getting better.'	Guilt, Frustration, Anger with self.
'What's the point? Maybe I should just accept that I'm going to be like this forever.'	Fear, Sadness, Hopelessness, Anger.
'I've done my best and it is not working.'	Frustration, Anger.
'Symptoms are a sign that some kind of damage is being done.'	Fear, Worry.

"This is just my life. I need to accept it."	Frustration, Anger.
"Why was I so stupid to think I could do …..?"	Frustration, Anger
"Maybe I am a normal person now." (when you get an increase in energy, which usually leads to overdoing it and a crash in energy).	False hope, hopelessness, Sadness

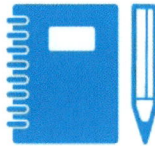

So, take some time to think about whether this sounds familiar to you. Have you slipped into a vicious cycle of draining emotions and avoidance or overdoing it? It is useful to become aware of your thoughts about coping and your actions to cope moving forward, so you can start to challenge some of these beliefs and behaviours during the process.

I also recommend that you listen to this video, which explains what happens at a biological level if we keep pushing our bodies over their limits on a regular basis:

Search: [Headington Institute: Unloading Allostatic Load - YouTube](#)

DISTURBED SLEEP PATTERNS

For many people who suffer from fatigue, getting good-quality and undisturbed sleep can feel like an uphill struggle. However, sometimes we let ourselves slip into unhealthy sleeping patterns over a period of time, and it's important to look at whether improving your sleep routine may be helpful in improving your symptoms and feelings towards your fatigue. So, why is sleep an important factor in managing fatigue?

Having very irregular bedtimes, getting up at different times each day or napping/resting excessively during the daytime can make it harder to fall asleep and stay asleep at night. This can lead to shortened sleep or can cause your sleep to be disturbed. Therefore, you will be unlikely to feel refreshed when you wake in the morning. This can trap you into a cycle of napping during the day because you're tired, then sleeping poorly again at night, and repeating the process. These types of disturbed sleep patterns can increase your feelings of fatigue. They can also lower your mood, worsen your symptoms or negatively impact the way you perceive your fatigue.

As you can see, sleep is an important factor to consider when managing your fatigue. So, I have included a space in your diary to record how much sleep you get day to day. This will help you to make links between the intensity of your symptoms and the amount and quality of sleep you are getting.

SYMPTOM FOCUSING

The symptoms commonly experienced by people with fatigue are both distressing and debilitating. So, it's completely understandable that you may spend a lot of time focusing on your symptoms. However, spending too much time paying attention to how you are feeling can make you feel them more intensely. This can also cause stress, which can exacerbate your symptoms further. Therefore, focusing on symptoms can heighten feelings of fear over carrying out activities that make you feel fatigued and can cause further avoidance.

LIFE STRESS AND LOW MOOD

Living with chronic fatigue can be extremely stressful, because the symptoms you experience affect the way you live your life day to day. Your illness may present you with various problems, including financial difficulties, concerns about being able to hold down a job or keep up with your studies. Many people with ongoing and debilitating fatigue may find that they are unable to socialise as much as they would like or in the way they want to so this can lead to giving up or avoiding socializing. It can become too exhausting to talk to people and deal with their questions.

Over time though this can lead to feelings of isolation and loneliness. For some people, they have been high achievers for most of their life, and they are used to operating at a fast pace. Life with CFS is a striking difference, which can cause low mood. Low mood can lead to a variety of problems, including tiredness, which can further reduce the desire to be active. As I discussed earlier, reducing activity levels too much can cause worsening of your condition over time.

It's also important to understand that stress and low mood can exacerbate your symptoms and can make your fatigue more intense. Therefore, monitoring your mood and stress levels is an extremely important part of the journaling process.

THE PHYSICAL AND MENTAL TOLL OF PERFECTIONISM

Perfectionism, a constant unrealistic, unforgiving striving for the unattainable can take its toll on you both mentally and physically. It can lead to isolation and disappointment and make you prone to getting sick and tired.

People with a tendency towards perfectionism tend to engage in 'all or nothing' thinking. This is a way of interpreting situations that is often referred to as being very 'black or white'. Therefore, your feelings about a certain situation will fall at one of two extreme ends of a spectrum. You have either succeeded totally or failed entirely. A task or activity either went perfectly, or it was a disaster. Everything has to be or look a certain way. This swaying between two extremes of emotions can be exhausting at a physical level and mental level.

Consider the example of an exam. You have completed most of the questions, then you arrive at a problem that you know you have revised but cannot remember the solution to. Your time is up, but you have still not answered that one question. Therefore, you consider yourself a failure, overlooking the fact that your overall performance on the paper was very good. For people who err towards this type of thinking, it can be hard to settle for something being 'good enough'.

Just as personality can be a factor in contributing to the development of fatigue, it can also be a perpetuating factor. People with a tendency towards perfectionism may be particularly prone to falling into unhelpful ways of managing their fatigue. Perfectionist personalities are more likely to find it difficult to take breaks and rests during the day, as they feel they are 'wasting time' and 'should be doing something useful'. However, planning a healthy level of rest into the day is not in fact wasting time at all. Instead, it is a vital part of managing your fatigue so you can continue to enjoy activities in a way that is sustainable.

This type of thinking can lead you to adopt the 'boom or bust' cycle of behaviour that I described earlier, where you engage in periods of intense activity followed by extended rest because you feel so exhausted. This is counterproductive, as it makes it difficult to establish a healthy routine, which is such an important part of positive management of your symptoms.

Perfectionism usually stems from an unhelpful deep rooted belief about yourself such as 'I'm unlovable', 'I'm not worthy', 'I'm not good enough' or 'I'm second best.' You may not be aware of these beliefs, but they drive your thinking style and behaviour. People engage in perfectionism as a way to hide these deep beliefs. The problem is that the reality is you can't be perfect 100% of the time, when you are in a situation where you can't be perfect this can cause anxiety or low mood as you evaluate the situation in accordance with your unhelpful deep beliefs about yourself, after some time, you start to think that the way forward is to perfect your perfectionism, in other words, you need to become better at being perfect. Over time, you have put unrealistic demands upon yourself and your everyday state becomes one of exhaustion. This pattern has been termed 'The perfectionist trap.'

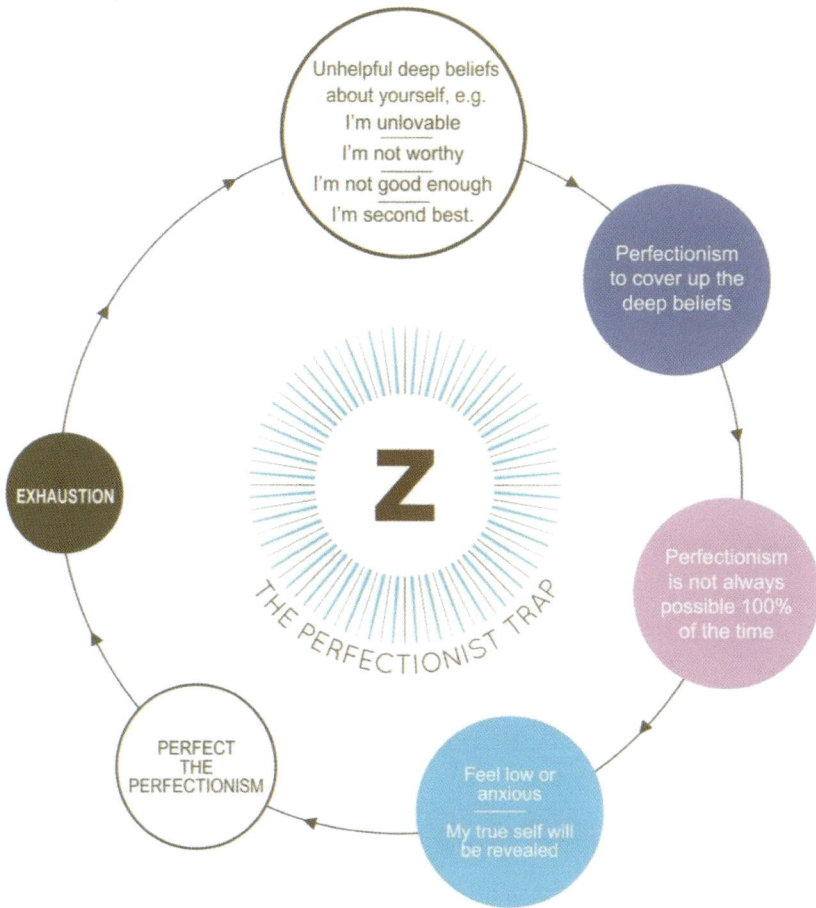

THE PERFECTIONIST TRAP

Unhelpful deep beliefs about yourself, e.g.
I'm unlovable
I'm not worthy
I'm not good enough
I'm second best.

Perfectionism to cover up the deep beliefs

Perfectionism is not always possible 100% of the time

Feel low or anxious
My true self will be revealed

PERFECT THE PERFECTIONISM

EXHAUSTION

This image is available at:

https://www.zenitudeselfhelp.com

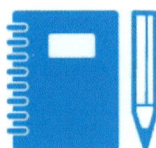

If this sounds like you, don't worry. Simply be aware that you tend towards this pattern of thinking as you progress through the book. Try to notice if you fall into perfectionist thinking so you can begin to challenge some of your less helpful beliefs, especially around rest. Make a note of any extreme language you use such as "Never" "Always" "Totally" "Total disaster" "There was no point at all" "What a total waste of time."

WORRY

Mind chatter can be exhausting. As with any long-term illness, anxiety is common in people living with chronic fatigue. As fatigue can have far-reaching effects on your life, it's only natural that this can cause distress and anxiety. Anxiety may be related to concerns about your health and the fear of worsening symptoms or pain. You may also be struggling with financial concerns, problems with interpersonal relationships or worries about how to cope with your illness at work.

USING YOUR DIARY

Now that you are aware of the factors that can impact fatigue, it is time to start a diary to honestly reflect on your own experience of fatigue and to pay attention to trying to understand your body, your thoughts and your behaviours.

Before you begin your diary work, it is a good idea to practice the following mindfulness technique. This will place you in the best possible mindset to begin making these links and connections. During this exercise, you will be paying attention to your posture. In particular, you will be noticing whether your posture is alert or not alert. When you are in an alert posture, you will be sitting upright in an engaged position. Slumping or slouching in your chair indicates that your posture in non-alert.

INSTRUCTIONS

1. Sit down somewhere comfortable and peaceful where you will not be disturbed. Close your eyes.
2. Turn your attention towards your posture. Is it an alert or non-alert position?
3. Notice how it feels to be sitting in your chair, right now. Pay attention to how your feet feel on the floor, your clothes against your skin, and where your weight is placed. The purpose of this exercise

is to develop a greater level of awareness of your body, not about making judgements on yourself. Try to let go of any judging thoughts.

4. After a few minutes, and when you feel ready, stop and note down any observations in your diary. What physical sensations did you notice?

Now you've set yourself up to notice how you are feeling in both body and mind, it's time to fill in your daily diary entry. Using the structured diary will prompt you to record all the information you need to start making links between key factors such as sleep, mood and activity levels and your symptoms.

The following diary pages are available for download at:

https://www.zenitudeselfhelp.com

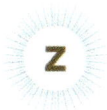

DAILY DIARY

TO BECOME IN TUNE WITH YOUR MIND & BODY

DAY: DATE: TIME: HOURS SLEPT LAST NIGHT:

ACTIVITY - What are you doing?

MOOD - How would you describe your mood?

THOUGHTS - What are you thinking about how you are coping?

What are you thinking about your fatigue?

BODY
ENERGY LEVELS   ①   ②   ③   ④   ⑤   ⑥   ⑦   ⑧   ⑨   ⑩
Rate intensity 0 - 10

BODILY FEELINGS - Notes on symptoms improvement or worsening

DAY: DATE: TIME: HOURS SLEPT LAST NIGHT:

ACTIVITY - What are you doing?

MOOD - How would you describe your mood?

THOUGHTS - What are you thinking about how you are coping?

What are you thinking about your fatigue?

BODY
ENERGY LEVELS   ①   ②   ③   ④   ⑤   ⑥   ⑦   ⑧   ⑨   ⑩
Rate intensity 0 - 10

BODILY FEELINGS - Notes on symptoms improvement or worsening

DAY:	DATE:	TIME:	HOURS SLEPT LAST NIGHT:

ACTIVITY - What are you doing? _____

MOOD - How would you describe your mood? _____

THOUGHTS - What are you thinking about how you are coping? _____

What are you thinking about your fatigue? _____

BODY ENERGY LEVELS
Rate intensity 0 - 10

① ② ③ ④ ⑤ ⑥ ⑦ ⑧ ⑨ ⑩

BODILY FEELINGS - Notes on symptoms improvement or worsening _____

_____

_____

_____

_____

_____

DAY:	DATE:	TIME:	HOURS SLEPT LAST NIGHT:

ACTIVITY - What are you doing? _____

MOOD - How would you describe your mood? _____

THOUGHTS - What are you thinking about how you are coping? _____

What are you thinking about your fatigue? _____

BODY ENERGY LEVELS
Rate intensity 0 - 10

① ② ③ ④ ⑤ ⑥ ⑦ ⑧ ⑨ ⑩

BODILY FEELINGS - Notes on symptoms improvement or worsening _____

_____

_____

_____

Z

_____

DAY: DATE: TIME: HOURS SLEPT LAST NIGHT:

ACTIVITY - What are you doing? _____

MOOD - How would you describe your mood? _____

THOUGHTS - What are you thinking about how you are coping? _____

_____

What are you thinking about your fatigue? _____

_____

BODY ENERGY LEVELS
Rate intensity 0 - 10
(1) (2) (3) (4) (5) (6) (7) (8) (9) (10)

BODILY FEELINGS - Notes on symptoms improvement or worsening _____

_____

_____

_____

_____

_____

_____

DAY: DATE: TIME: HOURS SLEPT LAST NIGHT:

ACTIVITY - What are you doing? _____

MOOD - How would you describe your mood? _____

THOUGHTS - What are you thinking about how you are coping? _____

_____

What are you thinking about your fatigue? _____

_____

BODY ENERGY LEVELS
Rate intensity 0 - 10
(1) (2) (3) (4) (5) (6) (7) (8) (9) (10)

BODILY FEELINGS - Notes on symptoms improvement or worsening _____

_____

_____

_____

_____

_____

Z

INSTRUCTIONS

ACTIVITY - *Note what you have been doing during the 3 hour period.*
Be specific with your descriptions of what you did. For example, if you said 'stayed at home'. What did you do? An example might be 'watched TV on the sofa' 'spoke to friend on the telephone' 'washed up'.

MOOD - *Describe how you felt.*
Rate your feeling on a scale of 1 to 10, with 1 being the least intensity of feeling and 10 being the most.

Here is a list of common moods that may help you:

SADNESS	GLAD	ANGER	ANXIOUS
EMBARRASSED	PLEASED	RAGEFUL	FEARFUL
SHAMED	HAPPY	FURIOUS	SCARED
DESPAIRING	JOYFUL	CROSS	TERRIFIED
MELANCHOLY	ELATED	VEXED	NERVOUS
BLUE	EXCITED	INCENSED	APPREHENSIVE
GLOOMY	PASSIONATE	IRATE	ALARMED

THOUGHTS - *Pause and think what has been going through your mind.*
Have you been worrying about anything? What have you been thinking about your fatigue? Is it annoying you? Are you worrying about the future? Are you thinking about things you can't do anymore? Are you thinking about different ways to try to deal with your fatigue? Note any thoughts of words that have come to mind in the past 3 hours. Take your time to work this out.

BODY ENERGY LEVELS - *Rate your energy levels on a scale of 0 - 10.*
0 = complete 'rust-out', tired from doing nothing, 5= enough energy to carry out your day as planned. 10= exhausted from having done too much.

BODILY FEELING - *How does your body feel?*

Here is a list of words that may help you to tune into what is going on in your body.

ACHY	DIZZY	JUMPY	SPINNING
BLOATED	DULL	LIGHT	STRONG
BLOCKED	ELECTRIC	NAUSEOUS	SUFFOCATING
BREATHLESS	ENERGIZED	NUMB	SWEATY
BUBBLY	EXPANSIVE	POUNDING	TENSE
BUZZY	FLUSHED	PRESSURE	THICK
CHILLS	FLUTTER	PRICKLY	THROBBING
CLAMMY	FRANTIC	PUFFY	TIGHT
COLD	FROZEN	RADIATING	TINGLY
CONGESTED	FUZZY	SHAKY	TREMBLING
CONSTRICTED	HEAVY	SHARP	WARM
DENSE	ITCHY	SMOOTH	WATERY

SYMPTOM NOTES - Think about anything you have noticed that may have made your symptoms worse or better. For example, did you walk too much? Did you go out for a walk and feel energized?

60

Phase 3 - Optimize your coping style and energy levels

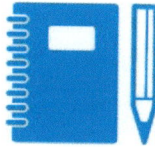

Find time to sit somewhere quiet and ask yourself 'What have I noticed from my diary?' Write down your observations.

Don't jump into making any changes all at once. Read the following techniques, then plan where you are going to start. Working with a psychologist would help you to pace you through your changes and support you to take realistic and incremental steps, working through any setbacks with you along the way. Talking through your plan of change with someone you trust will help to give you some perspective on the realistic nature of your plan. Also it usually helps to enhance your commitment to change once you have shared it with someone out loud.

As we move into this phase, we will be focusing on reframing your thought patterns and behaviour to start making positive changes to your routine. However, don't put down your diary just yet! It's important to keep monitoring your activity and fatigue levels throughout the process so you can spot patterns and figure out what works for you. None of the techniques are stand-alone techniques that are going to work in isolation. To make improvements to your fatigue levels, you really need to have done the diary work and to understand what is going on for you and what you need.

DEALING WITH UNHELPFUL THINKING PATTERNS ABOUT FATIGUE

It may sound too simple to notice and rethink your thoughts about fatigue. You may say, *how can something so simple help me?* You may feel outraged by the suggestions of something so simple. Well, it looks simple on paper, but the practice of noticing your thoughts, rethinking them repetitively is not simple. It does take patience, insight and effort. At first, the new ways of thinking may not seem real at all. I urge you to give it some time, and gradually you will notice some difference. To encourage you to continue, please pay attention to how you feel when you start to change your way of thinking.

Fatigue is real and it is not all in your head, but all the questions you may have may feel like it is a head experience. Quite often, my clients get stuck on the following thoughts: 'why?'

'why me?'

'why now?'

'why not her or him?'

'why can't I fix this?'

Do you hear yourself saying this? If so, notice the tone of your voice. Is this a kind or helpful voice? Probably not. It is more likely to be harsh, cold or angry. Thinking about who that voice reminds you of can be quite motivating to want to change that voice.

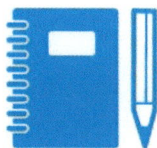

Next time you hear that harsh, cold or angry tone as you think about your fatigue, ask yourself:

Does the voice remind me of anyone in my past who was critical of me?

Write the name of that voice in your notebook.

My critical voice belongs to..............

Of course, as there is often no clear medical reason for your fatigue, it's only natural to wonder why this has happened to you, and it can all seem very unfair.

First, I would try to encourage you to have some compassion for your sick body. Fatigue is a human experience. Humans get sick and experience pain. It is not our fault that we get ill. It is part of the human bodily experience. I know when clients have become more compassionate towards their body, as I hear a sigh of relief. Listen to your breath and your body as you start to engage with it more compassionately.

MORE COMPASSIONATE THOUGHTS INCLUDE:

"I know you are working hard, dear body. I appreciate all the work you are doing."

"Getting information about therapies or diets that don't work for me, is important data in a process of finding what does work for me."

"Being human means being imperfect. Everyone has some sort of painful experience."

"My body is not my enemy. We are on the same team."

"Why not me? Humans get sick."

"I can feel bad and still choose to take a new and healthy action."

"I don`t need to rush, I can take things slowly."

As you read this, do you notice a sign of relief? What happens to your body?

Here is another technique to enhance this practice:

Rub your hands together. Place your hands on the different parts of your body that are causing suffering.

Say:

"I forgive you, dear body, for causing this pain. We are on the same team. Let's work together."

Next, think about the parts of your body that are working well.

Rub your hands together. Place your hands on the parts of the body that are working well.

Say:

"Thank you, dear (name the part of the body, e.g. heart) for working well."

Frustration is understandable. Have you identified thoughts that make you frustrated? Are they similar to the examples that I have given, such as:

'I'm getting so much support and I'm not getting better.'

'What's the point? Maybe I should just accept that I'm going to be like this forever.'

'I've done my best and it is not working.'

Despite any frustration, we need to learn to forgive our bodies if they get sick. Recovery is a very personal journey and comparing yourself to others is not useful.

As fatigue can have far-reaching effects on your life, it's likely that you'll have many thoughts and feelings about your illness. Beliefs about fatigue can be deep-seated and can affect the way that we behave and manage the condition. So, it's important to examine and challenge these thoughts in more detail to decide if they are accurate and if they are helpful or unhelpful. As an example, many people hold the belief that taking part in activities will always make their symptoms worse. While they may experience worsening of symptoms after some types and intensities of activity, this can lead to avoidance which can hinder recovery. So, a belief that *any* level of activity will definitely lead to pain or increased fatigue is not necessarily helpful. As these thoughts arise, try using the following steps to examine their usefulness:

FIND EVIDENCE FOR AND AGAINST YOUR THOUGHTS

Using your personal experiences and the knowledge you have gathered from your own research and through reading this book, compile evidence both for and against your belief. This will help you to look at a potentially emotional subject in a more objective way. So, examples may include:

1. "If I take the kids to the park, all my energy would be used, so I had better stay at home."

2. This thought might make you feel sad, disappointed in yourself, and angry.

3. "It would take all my energy to invite our friends over at the weekend. I'd have to cook and clean,

which would take a whole day, then I would spend the next day recovering and the whole weekend would be gone. So, I had better not invite them."

4. This thought might make you feel upset, isolated and bored.

GENERATING ALTERNATIVE THOUGHTS

Now you have looked at your thought in more detail, ask yourself if there is an alternative thought you could replace your original one with, based on your objective evidence. For example: 'If I balance my activities with periods of rest, I can still do the things I want to do.'

In both the above examples of unhelpful thoughts, some absolute words and 'all or nothing' thinking are being used.

Absolute words in these examples include: "all my energy", "whole day, "whole weekend".

Think!

"Would it really use all your energy?"

"Would it really take your whole day or whole weekend?"

Are there any alternatives here rather than not doing the activity?

1. Could you sit on the bench in the park? Could you ask a friend to go with you to the park? Could you sit in the garden with the children?

2. Could you ask friends to bring the food? Could you use paper plates? Could you keep the meal simpler than you would normally? Could you ask friends to join in with the cooking and cleaning?

SEE WHETHER THE UNHELPFUL THOUGHT HAS BECOME A BIT MORE FLEXIBLE.

Once you have generated an alternative thought, go back to your original, unhelpful thought and see how you feel about it now. Do you believe it with the same conviction as before? Do you feel more aligned with your original thought or your new, alternative thought?

DEALING WITH PERFECTIONISM

During Phase 2, I explored perfectionist thinking and how it can impact the way you cope with your fatigue. If perfectionism is part of your personality, approach this aspect of your personality with understanding and compassion. We all have unique personalities, and perfectionism is a trait shared by many people. However, it is important to be mindful of your perfectionist streak and to challenge these types of thought patterns. This is because perfectionist thoughts can drive you to continue with intense activity or overdo your solution/cure seeking and avoid rest, because you feel you should always be doing something productive. However, appropriate rest is actually highly productive for those living with fatigue, because it will help you to continue your activities in a manageable way.

This type of thinking can derail your efforts to make positive changes, such as following a diet or exercise regime, or in our case, establishing healthy new thought patterns and routines. If you don't feel like you have performed perfectly, you may feel like you have failed entirely, and this can cause you to become demotivated and give up, and for some, to frantically search for the next new method.

The solution to this is to try to look at the 'bigger picture' and gain a more realistic and compassionate perspective on what you are really achieving. Instead of focusing on what has gone wrong, it's important to notice and congratulate yourself on the many things you have done right! Giving yourself permission to do things well enough instead of perfectly is a kinder and more realistic way of managing your fatigue. I have two helpful suggestions for how you can begin to manage perfectionist thinking to help you on your journey to living with fatigue in a more balanced way.

THE 80/20 RULE

An interesting and useful concept when dealing with perfectionism is the 80/20 rule, or Pareto's rule. When you regularly experience fatigue, you have a limited amount of energy to expend. When you consider the things that you feel you want to (or ought to) be doing, this can seem overwhelming in comparison to your activity threshold.

Pareto was an Italian economist who observed that 80% of land belonged to the wealthiest 20% of people. He then explored this further and discovered that the 80/20 rule applied to a wide variety of situations. It follows that 20% of your activities will lead to 80% of your productivity. In other words, this is a way of prioritising your activities to make your load more manageable.

Try writing out your to-do list in your diary. Remember to not just include chores or work-related tasks, but also leisure and social activities that bring you joy. Taking part in pleasurable activities will improve your mood and sense of well-being, and you deserve to make these a priority. Now, try writing these out in order of importance and mark out the top 20%. Try focusing on accomplishing the top 20% instead of getting bogged down in the 80% that are less vital. This will make your list of activities less overwhelming and will ensure that you are expending your limited energy on the things that matter most.

It may seem to you that there are items in your 80% that are still very important. Could you ask for help from family, friends or colleagues to accomplish these tasks to leave you free to focus on your top 20%?

AIM FOR EXCELLENCE AS OPPOSED TO PERFECTION

Many people see excellence and perfection as the same thing. However, in reality aiming for excellence in what you do is far more healthy, productive and rewarding than striving for perfection. So, how do the two differ?

Essentially, perfection is an unattainable standard that we aim for out of fear of not being good enough. When we fail to achieve this unreachable goal, the result is self-criticism and a sense of failure. Perfection means getting things right 100% of the time and achieving 100% of what we set out to do, which is a feat so unmanageable that even those with boundless energy would fail.

Excellence, however, means striving to do the best that *you* can do in your daily activities. It involves focusing on the tasks that really matter and aiming to get them done to a high standard, but not to a perfect standard. This is an achievable and aspirational aim and will be far better for your self-esteem and sense of achievement than constantly chasing perfection. If you apply Pareto's 80/20 rule, the aim of reaching excellence is a good fit. This means that in the time it would take you to try to carry out one task to complete perfection, you could achieve several other goals to an excellent standard in the same timeframe. Shifting your thinking in regard to what is an acceptable standard will free up your time and allow you to do more while expending less energy.

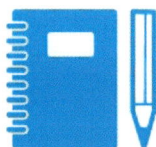

Think about how you use your time. Pick one thing you do to perfection and make a goal to do it to an excellent standard instead. What do you need to change? What do you need to stop doing? What do you need to stop thinking? What will be the worst thing that would happen if you make some changes?

KNOW YOUR DRAINERS AND ENERGIZERS

Have you noticed what and who drains your energy or energizers you? Do you have too many unfinished projects, unread books, cupboards that need tidying, clothes and gadgets you never use. Does a friend, family member of a colleague put too many demands on you? All of this clutter can slowly drain our energy and take up too much mental space and chip away at your everyday focus. Similarly, there are certain objects, activities and people that can give us energy.

Make a list of your drainers and energizers. Make a plan to make some small adjustments to gradually reduce the drainers from your life and bring in more of your energizers.

DEALING WITH ANXIETY AND WORRY

Some people are more pre-disposed towards anxiety than others, and it can feel like a difficult cycle to break. However, working to decrease your anxiety can help you to cope with your fatigue in several ways. First, no one likes to feel anxious. Anxiety is an unpleasant sensation, and by tackling it, you can work towards improving your mood. This will help you to cope better with the challenges you face as a result of your fatigue. Also, anxiety can absorb a lot of our energy that could be better used elsewhere and can wreak havoc with your all-important sleep patterns. So, you can see that dealing with anxiety is a key component of coping with fatigue.

In this section, I have two practical strategies to help you deal with your anxiety head-on and to allow you to move towards a calmer and more peaceful mindset.

THE WORRY TREE FOR PROBLEM SOLVING

Worrying thoughts are one of the most bothersome symptoms of anxiety. People who are anxious tend to spend a lot of time focusing on worrying. While you may believe that worrying helps you to avoid and solve problems, the truth is that excessive worrying is unhelpful and a drain on your mental energy.

The worry tree gives you a key strategy for coping with worrying thoughts as they arise. The tree differentiates between two common types of worries:

There are hypothetical worries, which occur when we get bogged down in the "what ifs" and focus on worst case scenarios. For example, you may have not received a phone call for a while from a loved one and wonder if they are seriously ill or have been involved in a terrible accident. This can be followed by intrusive and unwanted worries about what would happen if that really was the situation. These types of worries are often about things completely beyond our control and can lead us to believing that the scenario is more likely than it really is.

Current worries, on the other hand, relate to real problems that are happening now. These are within our control to influence. The worry tree gives you ways of dealing with the problem instead of simply worrying about it, helping you to regain a sense of control and therefore reducing anxiety.

This image is available at:

https://www.zenitudeselfhelp.com

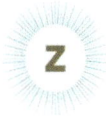

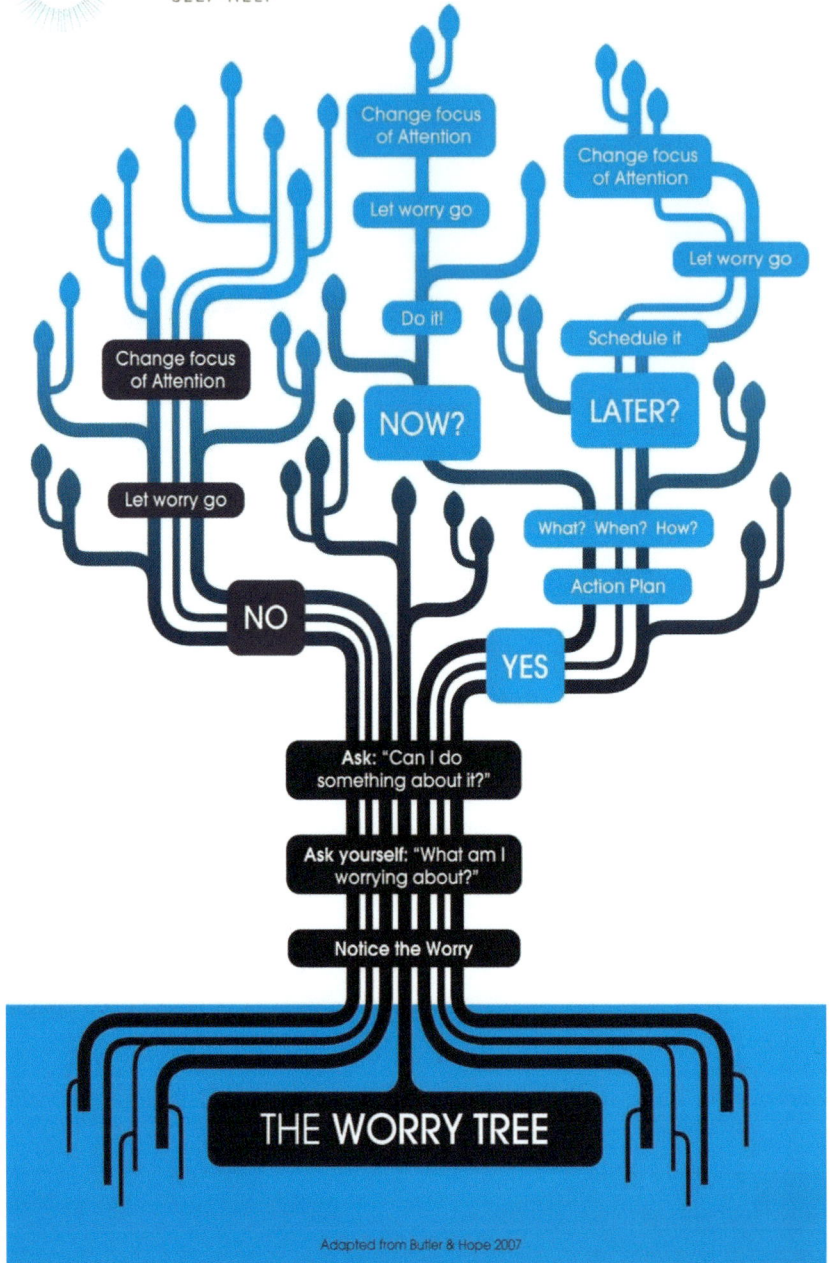

process into the following steps:

The first step is to notice that you are worrying and to clearly determine what you're worried about. For example, you may be worrying about a difficult financial situation or concerned that your bus is late and that you may be in trouble with your boss. Try to decide whether this is a current problem (the financial situation) or a hypothetical situation (being late and being fired). Also, ask yourself whether there is anything you can practically do to influence the situation.

IF YOU DECIDE YOUR CONCERN IS HYPOTHETICAL:

If your worry is hypothetical, then this means there is very little you can do about the situation. You can either choose to let go of your feelings of anxiety or come back to the worry at a later point. Whichever you decide, find something else to focus on to direct your thoughts away from the worry.

IF THE WORRY IS A CURRENT ISSUE:

Current problems are those that can be tackled through positive action. It's time to plan how you will tackle the problem to help alleviate your worry. Brain-storm a range of solutions. Don't think about the effectiveness of the solutions just yet. Just list possible solutions. Then look at the clearly defined problem and ask yourself, will the proposed solution help the defined problem. Choose the best solution first and plan a specific time to deal with it. Until that time, let go of your concern and find something else to do to shift your focus away from anxiety. If the first solution does not work, try the next solution.

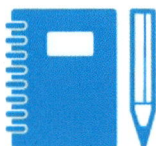

CIRCLES OF CONTROL AND INFLUENCE

People who suffer from ongoing fatigue have limited amounts of energy to expend before they reach their personal limit. This also applies to mental energy, as strenuous mental exertion can also be exhausting. Understanding your circles of control and influence help you to differentiate between situations and problems that we can control, and ones that we have no reasonable way of influencing.

Draw 3 circles of control like the one in the diagram. Think about a situation that is bothering you.

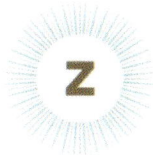

ZENITUDE
SELF-HELP

CIRCLE OF CONTROL

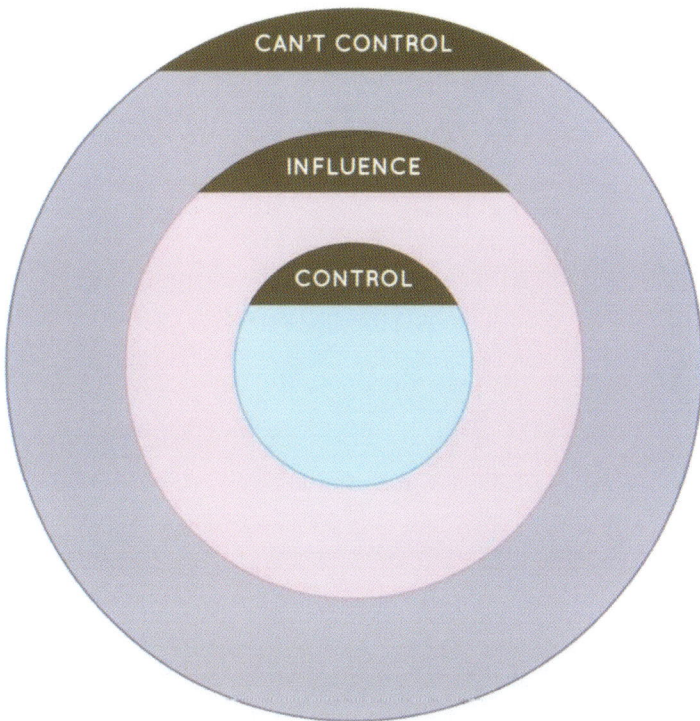

CAN'T CONTROL

INFLUENCE

CONTROL

This image is available at:

https://www.zenitudeselfhelp.com

The inner circle is that of control. You will probably have noticed that this is the smallest circle of all. That's because there are relatively few things that we have direct influence over. These are things such as our daily activities, when we go to bed, and what to eat for dinner.

The middle circle is the circle of influence. We don't have direct control over the problems or situations that fall in this circle; however, we can influence them in some way with our actions, although we cannot control them entirely. These could be things like how our kids achieve at school, what people think of us, or whether we are promoted at work.

The outer circle is the largest and the one we have the least control over. This is the circle of concern. This includes wider issues, such as terrorism or other current issues. While we may worry about these scenarios, there is no practical action that we can take to control them one way or the other.

The circles of control and influence are useful for helping us to decide whether something is worth expending our energy on. Try categorising your current concern into the circle where it fits best. If it falls into the inner circle, this is a situation you have direct control over. If the worry falls into the circle of influence, there may be something you can do to affect the outcome one way or the other. You will need to decide whether this is realistic and whether it is worth expending your energy on. If it is, you can make an action plan. If not, try to let go of the worry or postpone it to think about another time. Worries falling into the circle of control that are completely outside your influence may seem very concerning but it's important to accept that this is something you cannot control. When you find yourself worrying about these types of issues, try to refocus your mental energy elsewhere.

MINDFULNESS EXERCISE: LETTING GO OF WORRY AND VISUALISING THE WORRY GOING AWAY.

If you find yourself frequently worrying about hypothetical issues or concerns outside your circle of control, it's a good idea to try and let go of the worry. However, this can be easier said than done. If you are suffering from anxiety or are caught in a cycle of worry, simply releasing yourself from worry can be difficult to do. Try using this helpful mindfulness technique as a strategy for freeing yourself from worry over the things you can't control.

1. Sit in a comfortable position and either close your eyes or rest them gently on a fixed spot in the room.

2. Visualise yourself sitting beside a gently flowing stream with leaves floating along on the surface of the water. Pause 10 seconds.

3. .For the next few minutes, take each thought that enters your mind and place it on a leaf... let it float by. Do this with each thought – pleasurable, painful, or neutral. Even if you have joyous or enthusiastic thoughts, place them on a leaf and let them float by.

4. If your thoughts momentarily stop, continue to watch the stream. Sooner or later, your thoughts will start up again. Pause 20 seconds.

5. Allow the stream to flow at its own pace. Don't try to speed it up and rush your thoughts along. You're not trying to rush the leaves along or "get rid" of your worries. You are allowing them to come and go at their own pace.

6. If your mind says, "This is dumb," "I'm bored," or "I'm not doing this right," place those thoughts on leaves too, and let them pass. Pause 20 seconds.

7. If a leaf gets stuck, allow it to hang around until it's ready to float by. If the thought comes up again, watch it float by another time. Pause 20 seconds.

8. If a difficult or painful feeling arises, simply acknowledge it. Say to yourself, "I notice myself having a feeling of boredom/ impatience/ frustration". Place those thoughts on leaves and allow them to float along.

9. From time to time, your thoughts may hook you and distract you from being fully present in this exercise. This is *normal.* As soon as you realise that you have become side-tracked, gently bring your attention back to the visualisation exercise.

If you're used to routinely worrying, especially about things outside your control, letting go of your worries may not come naturally. That's okay. However, don't give up. By using this exercise on a regular basis, you will eventually come to terms with letting go of worry, and the process will become gradually easier. As you do the exercise, focus on how the worry makes you feel. Worrying is unpleasant, and the feelings associated with it will almost always be negative. Place these feelings on a leaf as well and send them away, replacing them with a more energetic feeling.

Tackling over-worrying is really worth your while, especially if you suffer from fatigue and associated muscle soreness and weakness. In fact, studies have found that the more anxious and stressed people are, the more tense and constricted their muscles become. Of course, I am not suggesting that your muscle pain or fatigue is caused by stress. Muscular fatigue or weakness is a common symptom associated with chronic fatigue. However, excessive stress or worry can make it worse. As you start to let go of your worries, I suggest you focus on your muscles. What happens to your body as you let go of your worry and stress?

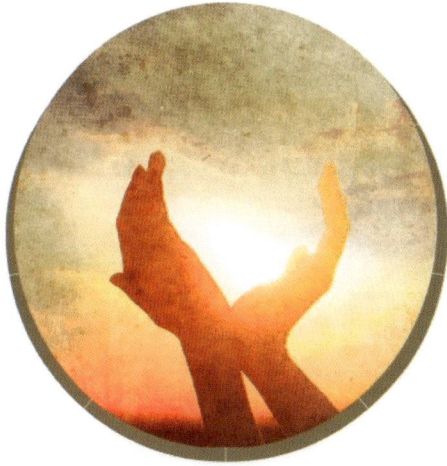

DEALING WITH CONCENTRATION DIFFICULTIES

Concentration difficulties can often be an issue associated with chronic fatigue. As you have limited energy to expend, and may also be struggling with anxiety, pain, or sleep problems, it's only natural that you may find focusing on tasks or thoughts difficult. It's also completely natural that you may want to take steps to improve your focus and concentration. This can help you to carry out your job more effectively or fully focus on and enjoy your everyday activities.

FLASHLIGHT TECHNIQUE

A practical technique I often recommend to my clients to improve their concentration is the flashlight technique. Try visualising a flashlight that you can adjust shining from the middle of your forehead, where you can control the intensity and broadness of the beam. When you need to focus, imagine this as your 'beam of concentration'.

You could decide to shine the light over a wide area, taking in a lot of information about your surroundings at once. Or, you may wish to pinpoint the beam on a small area, like a spotlight. You can also shine your beam of concentration inside yourself to examine your thoughts and feelings broadly or in sharp focus. Using the flashlight technique, over time you will be able to control and focus your own beam of concentration more effectively.

STAY HYDRATED

Make sure your brain does not dry out. A 2% decrease in hydration can lead to a 20% loss in energy and the ability to think correctly.

How do you like to drink water?

If you don't like water, add some flavour. Try some vegetable or fruit slices, or herbs, such as mint or basil. Remember, good nutrition is also important for concentration and cognitive fitness.

If you like cold water, do you have enough available? Do you think to buy a jug or bottle for the fridge?

Are you in the habit of taking water with you when you leave your home? If not, what do you need to do to make this a habit?

If you like apps to track your health, there are some apps available that help you to keep track of your water consumption.

CREATE A TO-DO LIST FOR YOUR DISTRACTION

We live in a world where we can have access to information the second a mental request crosses our mind. As a result, many people toggle away from what they are working on the instance a thought about needing more information pops into their mind. The problem with this is that, once you are distracted, it takes an average of 25 minutes to return to the original task. Also, shifting your attention back and forth drains its strength.

To stay focused, whenever something pops into your head, just write it down on a piece of paper next to you or on an electronic note. Tell yourself you will look at this when you take a break from what it is you are trying to focus on. You can then evaluate the distraction To-Do list and ask yourself if it is still worthy of some attention and time.

DEALING WITH SLEEP PROBLEMS

Sleep problems are commonly experienced alongside fatigue. This can be exacerbated if you are experiencing painful symptoms or are worrying a lot. Also, if you find yourself sleeping for long periods during the day, this can make falling and staying asleep at night very difficult. However, trying to establish healthy sleeping habits and routines is very important. Disordered routines will make achieving good-quality sleep and waking feeling refreshed and re-energised practically impossible. However, by taking some practical measures, you can take your first steps towards more healthy and energising sleep habits. Here are my top strategies for establishing good sleeping patterns:

- Try to let go of worries before you go to sleep. If you have anxious thoughts whirring around your brain, it can be near-impossible to nod off quickly. So, it's a good idea to try to deal with worries at least an hour before you settle down. Schedule some 'worry time'. Use the Worry Tree to help you deal with your worries.

- If you don't have the time to deal with worries before bed, consider jotting down your worries in a notebook and tell yourself you will come back to them in the morning.

- If you find yourself still thinking before bed, repeat the word 'the' in your head and tell yourself that night-time is for sleep and that the brain is less effective at dealing with worries at night. The word 'the' is a boring and meaningless word that will suppress your unhelpful thoughts.

- Establish a regular sleep routine. Irregular bedtimes and waking times can make it difficult to sleep through the night. Although it may seem hard, try to go to bed and wake up at the same time every day, including at the weekends. Over time, your body will adjust to this new routine and you will be more likely to feel sleepy at bedtime.

- Avoid substances that could interfere with your sleep, especially in the afternoons and before bed. These include alcohol, nicotine and caffeinated beverages and foods.

- Don't stay in bed if you can't sleep. You want your body to associate your bed with sleeping so that it is ready to fall asleep when you settle down for bed. For this reason, it's also a good idea not to watch TV or carry out any other activities whilst lying in bed. If you can't sleep, get up and take part in a calming activity, such as reading for a while, until you feel ready to nod off.

DEALING WITH LOW MOOD AND DEPRESSION

Many people with fatigue develop feelings of depression and low mood. Depression can also affect the way you experience fatigue, making your symptoms more intense. Many people find it difficult to ask for help with dealing with depression, but it is not a sign of weakness at all. In fact, depression is a common mental illness and could strike anybody at any time. It does not denote any kind of lack of strength or determination, and if you are struggling with depression, you deserve the help you need to feel better.

Some thinking styles are commonly shared amongst people with depression. Perfectionist style 'black and white' thinking, focusing on hypothetical worries, and assuming the worst are all common thinking styles when you're suffering from depression. If you recognise these thinking patterns in yourself, it's important to acknowledge and challenge them. Here is an example of how you can start to challenge one of these unhelpful thinking patterns.

ALL OR NOTHING THINKING STYLE

This type of thinking is particularly associated with depression. It is the tendency to think in terms of binary oppositions, such as "good" or "bad", "black" or "white", "healthy" or "unhealthy". This kind of thinking is quite rigid and can cause frustration and disappointment. Being frustrated and disappointed on a regular basis zaps your energy levels.

Ask yourself:

What is in the middle?

What am I not seeing/overlooking?

If I drew a scale from 0-100, what would be 75?

Dealing with depression requires help, understanding and support from others, and often from trained professionals. So, although it may feel hard, it's important to seek the help you need to begin to recover. While this may feel like admitting defeat, seeking support is a brave and courageous step. More and more people are seeking professional help for depression. Remember, you deserve support and compassion to help you get better. Take a moment to think about asking for help.

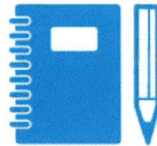

What do you think when you envision yourself asking for help? What do you feel in your body? Re-evaluate your thoughts by asking yourself, *what would I say to a friend who needed help?*

Does the feeling in your body when you think about asking for help, give you any clues?

DEALING WITH FOCUSING ON THE SYMPTOMS IN YOUR BODY

Often, we feel stress acutely in our bodies. This can be unpleasant and can also serve to worsen your fatigue symptoms. When you're suffering from stress in your life and are experiencing this in your body, you can try using the 'Soften, Soothe, Allow' technique to self-soothe.

Start by closing your eyes and focus on how you are feeling. What does that feeling need? How can you soothe the feeling?

SOFTEN

Once you have found the area of your body where you are experiencing the stress, begin by gently trying to soften the area, relaxing the muscles. If focusing on this area causes you discomfort, focus on your breathing until the sensation passes.

SOOTHE

Next, soothe yourself lovingly, because you are experiencing stress and discomfort. Direct kind and compassionate thoughts towards yourself and the area in which you are experiencing stress, tension or pain.

ALLOWING

Finally, allow and accept the discomfort to exist in you, allowing it to come and go naturally. Notice if your attention is too over-focused on these sensations. If so remind yourself that you have soothed your body, take a deep breath and change your focus of attention. It is good to think about when you tend to over-focus and pre-plan how you could change your focus of attention.

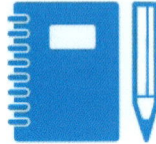

In your notebook, note the circumstances in which you over-focus on your body. Think of other things you could do in these circumstances to change your focus of attention.

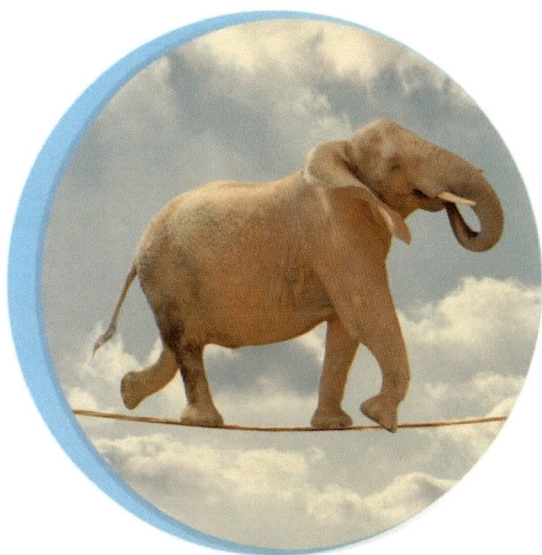

You may, as part of this process, need to get more active or reduce your activity. There will be times when you need to do more, and times when you need to rest.

There is some controversy about the benefits of adapting your activity levels. You must always consult your doctor to find out if this would be safe for you. Clients that I have worked with have benefited from pacing their activity levels. However, I suggest this is done with an increased body awareness. This takes time to understand your body and to know when it is ready to do a little more or when it has had enough.

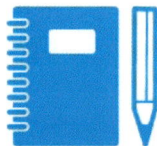

It is important to put some time into planning both activity and rest periods based on how your symptoms are affected and an awareness of your body. Think about what you have learnt from your diary work and put together a plan for both activity and rest periods. Start with what you would like your end goal to be, then think about your current levels of activities and rest. Then devise a plan with several steps that will take you closely to your goal. So, for example, if you find that you are waking up too late, then trying to work in the afternoon, but you find your energy levels dipping in the afternoon (most people tend to have energy dips around 3pm, it's part of the body's natural energy cycle). Suddenly waking up early is not realistic, so plan getting up 15 minutes earlier than normal for 3 days, then 30 minutes earlier than normal for the next 3 days. Continue in 15-minute decrements until you reach your goal.

Plan each day in advance and focus on activities that are realistic. You may need to adjust your expectations of what you can do based on what is *currently* realistic to you. I emphasize *currently*, as some people get so scared that this current level is fixed forever that they get tempted to force themselves to do more, as they don't want this *current* level to be forever. Forcing yourself beyond your *current* limit, however, will only put pressure on your body. So, when adjusting your expectations, do not base this on what you used to be able to do and wish you could still do. Tune into your *current* limits. This will change over time.

Over time, you will be able to modify and adapt your routine until you find a pattern of activity that is sustainable within your own energy limits and your knowledge of what does and does not exacerbate your symptoms.

A good way to plan your activity levels is to think of your energy reserves like a battery. If you burn through all your energy in one big burst, you will need longer to recharge. On the other hand, short and manageable periods of activity will require shorter, planned periods of 'recharging' to recover from. Therefore, it's important to pay close attention to the intensity and duration of your activity levels and how they affect your symptoms. Try and notice what your limit is before your symptoms are exacerbated. Gradually, you will learn how much activity you can endure comfortably without needing a long 'crashing out' period, and the frequency and duration of breaks you need to plan into your day. You may also find that you can manage more activity than you previously thought possible if you plan your activities around your limits carefully.

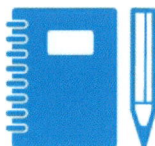

Now, you should have some insights into what factors are contributing to your fatigue. It is time to plan your next steps to start dealing with your fatigue, dealing with one factor at a time.

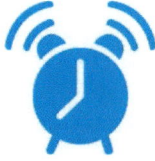

Write out your goals and give yourself some timeframes. Set some reminders for each goal. It can be tempting to try to fix everything at once. Please don't try this. It will create anxiety and cause further fatigue. For example you may have notice the following about yourself:

I use too much all or nothing thinking.

I worry too much.

I try too hard to get better.

I over-focus on my symptoms.

Look through the suggested ways of dealing with what has come up from you. Rate how doable each suggestion is for you on a scale of 1-5, with 1 being not very doable and 5 being doable. Start with the most doable, then when you feel you have made progress, start to think about the next goal on your list.

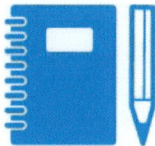

Before you start to make changes, think about what obstacles may prevent you from making the change, then brainstorm how you would overcome the obstacle. For example, you may recognize that you are too tired to cook healthy meals. What solutions are available to you? Write down as many ideas as possible then choose the best solution for you. So to continue with the example, you could plan some quick easy healthy options. It may mean changing what you consider to be healthy. It may mean taking it turns to batch cook with a friend. It may mean buying more frozen vegetables rather than fresh vegetables. It may mean preparing breakfast the night before. It may mean asking someone in the family to regularly chop up fruit and keep it in the fridge.

When you've worked through Phase 3, take a little time to look back over your progress and congratulate yourself on your successes.

Phase 4 – Living your Energized Life

The final phase in the process is to reflect on the ways that your fatigue affects you and to set out on a new and positive course where you can manage your fatigue as part of a fulfilling life. At the beginning of this book, you created a vision of a realistic and hopeful future you. Take a moment to reflect on this image now you've completed the subsequent phases. Is your vision the same? What has changed? Is that okay? During phase 4, you will use your notebook to reflect and set goals and strategies for achieving this new and redefined life.

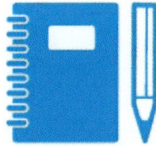

What has changed since you developed fatigue? What do you miss? What don't you miss? What have you learnt about yourself? Consider the following life areas while you reflect.

Work: Are you still working? Is your work impaired in any way? Have you given up everything else in order to maintain your career? If you're in work, ask yourself if you have a happy balance between work, activities that you enjoy, and rest.

Social: How has your social life changed? Has the type and frequency of your socialising changed, and how? Think about whether there have been any changes in the people you most frequently spend time with.

Sport/Activity: How has this changed? Is there anything you can't do now that you used to enjoy? Are there new things that you would like to try but feel unable to do so?

Home: Are you unable to clean, cook, care for the children etc.? If not, who is now doing the work? Are you happy with this? Do you want to make some changes?

Personal relationships: If you are in a relationship, how has this changed? It can sometimes be that the relationship gets stronger, on the other hand it can cause strain on both partners. What do you appreciate about this relationship? What do you want to change in this relationship? What is the first step you need to take? Do you need to stop doing something?

Family relationships: The dynamics can change within the family. This is more likely to happen in the case of there being a role reversal, e.g. the husband becoming the primary caregiver. If there have been big changes, how do you feel about them? People with fatigue can feel very guilty about not doing as much with or for their family as they used to do. Is the emotion draining you? Can you learn to rethink the draining emotion? Do you need to change what you are doing?

Finally, consider if there are any other factors that could be impacting on your fatigue. These could be social, physical, emotional or financial. What is your first step to changing these factors?

It's common to find that your interpersonal relationships have been impacted by your fatigue. If this is the case for you, now is a great time to begin developing strategies to help you deal with the important people and activities in your life. Honest and open communication is key. You may find it hard to explain to loved ones how you feel about your illness, but it's important to be able to talk about how fatigue has impacted your lives. Being able to listen to the viewpoints of your loved ones is also key. If you are struggling with your relationships, particularly with your spouse or partner, it may be worth seeking out specialist guidance to help you work through any issues in a safe and positive way.

Take a moment to think about what your new hopes are for the future. These could be related to your mood and feelings about your illness, your activity levels, symptoms, your relationships and interactions with others, your career or your passions/hobbies.

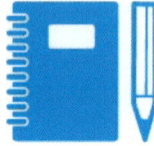

Jot down your redefined goals in your journal. Ask yourself: is there anything getting in the way of you achieving your goals?

Now, think about how you could overcome these obstacles and move towards achieving your aims. Trying to reach a goal in one big step can seem overwhelming. Instead, try to think about the small steps you will need to take to achieve each goal, and tackle them one step at a time. This will make the goal less overwhelming, especially as you are already suffering from fatigue. With a plan to make your goal achievable in manageable chunks, this makes success far more likely. Some people seek the help of a Coach to help them overcome obstacles for change.

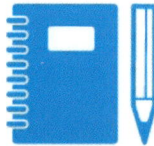

Finally, consider your personal qualities that will help you towards your desired outcomes. You are a unique individual with a unique set of strengths that you can draw upon as you work towards your new positive future. Perhaps you are resilient, kind or a good communicator? Make a list of the strengths you have in your toolkit that will allow you to succeed. Sometimes, it can be hard to see and recognise positive qualities in yourself. You may want to ask a trusted loved one who knows you well to help you with this exercise.

Look at the box of examples of strengths to help you define your strengths. Which strengths do you need to draw upon to continue to make progress?

EXAMPLES OF STRENGTHS

Sincere	Wise	Thoughtful
Calm	Organised	Creative
Patient	Positive	Generous
Determined	Dependable	Resilient
Appreciative	Engaging	Insightful
Warm	Humorous	Caring
Focused	Brave	Fair
Strategic	Rigorous	Independent

Understanding	Detailed	Hopeful
Open-minded	Practical	Playful
Curious	Supportive	Decisive

FINALLY

As discussed, fatigue can be a debilitating illness and can have distressing and life-changing effects. Unfortunately, I cannot claim to cure the root causes of your fatigue, if there is an underlying disease. However, hopefully you have seen, while reading this book, that you can make positive changes to your mindset, routine and activity levels to make living with fatigue more manageable. In some cases, these exercises are enough to eliminate the feelings of fatigue.

The process of dealing with fatigue does not stop here. Throughout this book, I have introduced you to a series of useful exercises and techniques to help you manage stress, anxiety and tension. You may find it helpful to revisit these whenever you are experiencing periods of increased symptoms, stress or worry.

By completing the process in this book, you have taken great steps towards a more positive future. Changing deeply ingrained habits and ways of thinking is never easy, but I believe the effort will pay dividends in terms of stress and anxiety reduction, improved sleep quality, and more effective symptom management. Remember to take time to be kind and compassionate towards yourself and to congratulate yourself on the progress you have made so far.

About the Author

Hi, I established Zenitude Self Help. I want to reassure you that I have the necessary expertise and experience to help you. I'm a Chartered Psychologist and a Cognitive Behavioural Therapist. I've dedicated my whole career to researching and practising psychology. I have spent many years helping thousands of people to become happier, healthier and more successful.

I am the author of the Amazon bestselling book, 'Slim Mind' which was ranked as number 1 in the Cognitive Behavioural Therapy (CBT) category. I have spent many years researching how CBT can improve lives. I have contributed to the scientific evidence for the effectiveness of CBT in numerous scientific journals and books.

As well, I have presented my evidence at scientific conferences. Mixed with my expertise, I am passionate about psychology and its potential to help people lead happier and healthier lives. Over the years I have seen how much of a change can be made by psychological approaches and I would like to help more people access that change. It is common for psychologists to practice one approach. However I believe that by combining all the best aspects of what psychology has to offer that a fuller method can be provided.

In my Zenitude series I dare to mix up psychological approaches to bring you tools and techniques that help address issues from a wider psychological perspective. Therefore you will find CBT, Acceptance and Commitment Therapy (ACT), Mindfulness and hypnosis techniques as well as influences from Somatic Psychology in my programmes. I truly hope you will take away useful techniques to improve your life.

Dr Catherine Sykes

ZENitudeselfhelp.com

All of the illustrations and material in this book are available at ZENitudeselfhelp.com

You can also find out more about booking a one-to-one therapy or coaching on-line session at ZENitudeselfhelp.com

You can also find out more about becoming a reviewer of other self-help books in the ZENitude Self Help Series at ZENitudeselfhelp.com

Also check out the Zenitude FACEBOOK page for regular inspiration and support.

facebook.com/zenitudeselfhelp/

Printed in Great
Britain
by Amazon